HERBS FOR POISON AND INSECT BITES

Harnessing Nature's Healing Power, A Guide To Treating Poisonous Exposures And Stings With Nature's Bounty

DR. JEREMY ALLEY

Disclaimer:

The information provided in this book, is intended for general informational purposes only and should not be considered as professional advice.

The author has made every effort to ensure the accuracy of the information presented. However, readers are advised to consult with a qualified healthcare professional before attempting any herbal remedies or making significant changes to their wellness routine. Individual health conditions vary, and what may be suitable for one person may not be appropriate for another.

It is important to note that the author is not in any endorsement deal, partnership, or affiliation with any organization, brand, or company mentioned in this book. Any references to specific products or services are based on the author's personal experience or general knowledge and do not imply an endorsement or promotion of those products or services.

Contents

Overview

Herbal treatments are well known in the field of natural medicine for their ability to treat a wide range of medical issues. This includes how well they work to lessen the pain brought on by poison and bug stings. This guide examines the use of herbal treatments in certain circumstances and offers information on their uses and advantages.

About This Book

Traditional medicine has a long history of using plants and their extracts for medicinal purposes, which led to the development of herbal treatments. Herbal remedies provide a comprehensive method of treating the symptoms of poisoning and insect bites. Several plants have anti-inflammatory, antiseptic, and calming ingredients that can help lessen the effects of venom or toxins ingested through bites.

Calendula, chamomile, and lavender are among the well-known herbs for their calming and anti-inflammatory qualities. For example, calendula is a wonderful addition to herbal remedies for bites because it contains therapeutic components that may help reduce inflammation and stimulate skin regeneration. Because of its relaxing qualities, chamomile can help reduce the inflammation and itching that come with bug bites. Because of its antibacterial properties, lavender may help keep infections from growing at the bite site.

The Value of Herbal Remedies for Insect and Poison Bites

Herbal remedies for poison and insect bites are significant because they provide a safe, all-natural substitute for pharmaceutical ones. Herbal medicines frequently have fewer negative reactions than some pharmaceutical options, which makes them ideal for people with sensitivities or allergies.

Furthermore, people looking for an affordable and practical way to ease the discomfort caused by bites might choose herbal remedies, which are simple to create at home. People are empowered by this accessibility to take charge of their health and look into natural options that fit with their values and interests.

Herbal medicines are also holistic, taking into account the patient's emotional and psychological well-being in addition to their physical ailments. Certain herbs have calming and soothing properties that support the mental resilience needed during the healing process and enhance general well-being.

Knowing the many advantages of using herbal remedies for poison and bug bites clarifies how important it is to include these non-prescription treatments in our healthcare regimen. Herbal remedies provide an effective and comprehensive way to deal with the pain and difficulties caused by poison and insect bites, whether they are employed as a first line of defense or in addition to traditional therapies.

Recognizing Insect Bite Hazards

Insect bites and poisonous interactions are frequent occurrences that can interfere with our everyday lives. Knowing what to look for in these situations is essential for timely and efficient treatment, whether the contact was caused by a toxic plant or a poisonous insect bite.

Typical Insects and Poisons

To treat poisoning and insect bites properly, one must become familiar with the typical offenders. Many plants, insects, and animals have poisons or venom that can cause negative reactions. Every encounter—from the infamous poison ivy to the deadly bites of spiders and snakes—needs a different strategy for treatment.

Symptoms and Reactions

It is essential to identify the reactions and symptoms of poisoning and insect bites to take prompt action. Depending on the particular poison or venom involved, symptoms can change. Redness, swelling, itching, and pain at the bite or exposure site are typical symptoms.

Severe cases may include breathing difficulties, nausea, or even anaphylaxis, which calls for emergency medical care.

Herbal remedies can be quite helpful in reducing symptoms and accelerating recovery from poisoning and bug bites.

For generations, people have relied on herbal treatments, which utilize the therapeutic qualities of different plants to alleviate the negative effects of poisoning and toxicity. Let's examine the herbal remedies that can be used to treat poison and insect bites in a safe, natural manner.

Herbal Remedies for Insect and Poison Bite Victims

Aloe Vera: Applied directly to the diseased area, aloe vera is well-known for its calming effects. It relieves the pain brought on by bites by reducing redness and swelling thanks to its anti-inflammatory and cooling properties.

Calendula: A valuable herbal medicine for poisoning and bug bites, calendula possesses anti-inflammatory and antibacterial qualities. To aid in healing, the damaged region can be treated with calendula creams or ointments.

Chamomile: Chamomile is a great option for reducing itching and irritation brought on by bites because of its relaxing and anti-inflammatory qualities. Compresses or lotions infused with chamomile can be soothing.

Echinacea: Well-known for strengthening the immune system, echinacea helps support the body's natural healing mechanism. Using lotions laced with echinacea or taking pills may help recuperation.

Lavender: Lavender essential oil offers calming and antibacterial qualities. To lessen inflammation and encourage healing, the afflicted region can be treated with diluted lavender oil.

Tea Tree Oil: Tea tree oil has antibacterial and anti-inflammatory qualities. It can be administered topically to the bite site after being diluted. It lessens edema and aids in infection prevention.

Even while herbal medicines are a great help in treating poisoning and insect bites, you should always seek expert medical attention, particularly in severe cases. These herbal remedies offer all-natural relief from common symptoms and can be used in conjunction with conventional therapies. Individual reactions to herbal therapies may differ, as with any medical issue, therefore speaking with a healthcare provider is advised for specific guidance.

CHAPTER ONE

HERBS' PART IN HEALTHCARE

For ages, traditional medicine in many countries has relied heavily on herbs as a natural remedy for a wide range of ailments. Herbal medicines have proven their efficacy in aiding healing and providing relief in cases of poisoning and bug bites. To fully utilize the healing potential of herbs, it is essential to comprehend the fundamentals of herbal medicine, how herbs interact with the body and safety considerations.

Fundamentals Of Herbal Medicine

Phytotherapy, botanical medicine, and herbal medicine are terms used to describe the use of plants and plant extracts for the prevention, treatment, or mitigation of a variety of medical diseases. Herbs are abundant in bioactive substances with therapeutic qualities. Alkaloids, flavonoids, terpenes, and essential oils are a few examples of these chemicals. These herbal ingredients have the potential to treat the body when used or ingested correctly.

Herbs' Effects On The Body

The way that herbs interact with the human body is a complicated process. Bioactive substances found in herbs can affect physiological processes. Anti-inflammatory herbs, for instance, can help lessen the pain and swelling brought on by insect bites, and herbs that are detoxifying can help remove toxins from poisons. Utilizing herbs for healing effectively requires an understanding of their individual qualities and mechanisms of action.

Herbs can be applied topically or used as teas, tinctures, poultices, or other modes of administration. The type of ailment and the intended result determine which approach is best. Topical treatments, including herbal poultices or salves, are frequently useful in offering fast relief and accelerating the healing process for poison and insect bites.

Safety Points To Remember

Although using herbal treatments is a natural alternative, care must be taken when using them, particularly in cases of poisoning and insect bites. Certain herbs may cause allergies in certain people, and improper use or dosage may have negative effects. It is best to speak with a licensed herbalist, naturopath, or other healthcare provider, especially if there are any drugs or pre-existing medical issues involved.

Furthermore, correctly identifying herbs is essential to prevent utilizing harmful plants that could make the problem worse. For herbal use to be safe and successful, it is essential to educate oneself on the unique qualities of each herb and any potential interactions. Even when herbal therapies are included in the overall treatment plan, it is still necessary to seek emergency medical help in cases of serious poisoning responses, bug stings, or allergies.

Herbs are a great source of natural remedies for poisoning and insect stings. To fully utilize the healing power of these natural treatments, it is imperative to comprehend the principles of herbal therapy, how herbs interact with the body, and how to apply safety precautions.

CHAPTER TWO

BUILDING A FIRST AID KIT WITH HERBS

Making an herbal first aid box is a sensible first step toward natural and holistic healthcare, as herbs have been used for ages to manage a variety of health issues.

Herbal remedies can offer efficient relief and support for any type of injury, from a little bug bite to a more serious poison contact. This tutorial explains how to put together a portable herbal emergency kit and covers vital herbs for rapid reaction.

Crucial Herbs For Fast Reaction

Plantain: Well-known for its antibacterial and anti-inflammatory qualities, plantain is a useful herb for treating stings and bites from insects. Crushed leaves can be applied topically to ease discomfort and swelling.

Calendula: Calendula is useful for treating a variety of skin irritations, including bug bites, due to its antibacterial and anti-inflammatory properties. To aid in healing, apply a lotion or oil enriched with calendula to the injured region.

Aloe Vera: Known for its calming and cooling qualities, aloe vera gel works wonders for reducing the pain and swelling brought on by insect bites. Additionally, it aids in the skin's healing process.

Chamomile: Chamomile is a helpful herb for reducing itching and discomfort from insect bites because of its anti-inflammatory and soothing qualities. One can use chamomile tea topically or as a compress.

Lavender: The antibacterial and analgesic qualities of lavender essential oil are well known. Diluted lavender oil applied to insect bites helps avoid infection in addition to reducing discomfort.

Echinacea: Known for enhancing the immune system, echinacea supports the body's natural defenses following an insect attack when applied topically or orally.

It might aid in lowering inflammation and accelerating recovery.

Activated Charcoal: Adding activated charcoal to your herbal first aid kit can be quite helpful in cases of poisoning. It functions by attaching itself to toxins and stopping the bloodstream from absorbing them. Seek advice on its use from a healthcare expert at all times.

How To Assemble A Travel Herbal Kit

Think about the following advice when putting together a herbal first aid kit:

Compact Size: Make sure your emergency supply kit is small and lightweight, with only the necessities for rapid access in case of an emergency.

Storage Containers: For storing herbal preparations like tinctures, oils, and salves, choose compact, airtight containers. This keeps them from leaking and preserves their potency.

Labeling: Make sure to mark the name, uses, and expiration date of every plant and preparation. This guarantees efficient and safe use.

Add standard First Aid items: To address a variety of scenarios, carry standard First Aid items like bandages, tweezers, and scissors in addition to herbal medications.

You can be well-prepared to treat poison and insect bites with safe and efficient herbal remedies by including these necessary herbs and adhering to useful advice for assembling a portable kit.

CHAPTER THREE

HERBAL TREATMENTS FOR INSECT AND POISON BITES

It might be upsetting to deal with the fallout from poisoning or bug bites, but nature provides a variety of herbal medicines to ease pain and encourage recovery.

Plant-based Countermeasures: Several plants have natural defenses against poisons. Plantain (Plantago major) is one such noteworthy herb that is well-known for its capacity to counteract toxicity and lessen inflammation.

Crushed leaves can be applied topically to the afflicted area to relieve pain and irritation. Similarly, because of its anti-inflammatory components, jewelweed (Impatiens capensis) is known to be useful against oak and poison ivy.

Herbs known for their detoxification qualities can help cleanse the body and help get rid of toxic toxins.

The well-known detox herb dandelion (Taraxacum officinale) promotes liver function and aids in the body's effective removal of toxins. After being exposed to some chemicals or insect venom, dandelion tea or tincture made from it can help with the detoxification process.

Herbal Poultices and Compresses: By immediately applying the therapeutic qualities of herbs to the afflicted area, herbal poultices and compresses provide localized relief.

Because calendula (Calendula officinalis) has anti-inflammatory and wound-healing properties, it is frequently used in poultices. Calendula can be used to relieve irritation by combining it with a carrier oil and applying it to bites or stings. Comfrey (Symphytum officinale) is also prized for its capacity to encourage tissue healing, which makes it a useful ingredient in compresses for bites or small wounds.

Including these herbal remedies in your first aid kit can help treat poison and insect bites safely and efficiently.

Plant-based remedies, detoxifying herbs, or herbal compresses are just a few of the ways that nature provides for relieving the pain and fostering recovery related to these occurrences.

Herbal Remedies For Insect Bite Injury

Bites from insects can be uncomfortable, itchy, and inflammatory. Herbal treatments provide a safe, all-natural means of reducing these symptoms and encouraging recovery. Here, we look at several herbal remedies for insect bites, such as topical treatments, calming balms, and anti-inflammatory drinks.

Calm Herbal Balms

Herbal balms are a well-liked treatment for bug bites. Calendula, chamomile, and lavender are examples of ingredients with antibacterial and anti-inflammatory qualities. Particularly calendula is recognized for its ability to soothe skin, and chamomile relieves irritation. Lavender enhances the balm's overall relaxing impact and gives it a lovely scent. These herbs can be incorporated into a carrier oil and combined with beeswax to make a calming, skin-friendly salve that is known as an herbal balm.

Herbal Teas That Reduce Inflammation

In addition to being soothing to drink, herbal teas can be applied topically to treat insect bites. Yarrow, comfrey, and plantains are a few examples of herbs with anti-inflammatory qualities.

These dried herbs can be soaked in boiling water and then allowed to cool to make an herbal tea for insect bites.

Next, using a fresh towel or cotton ball, apply the resulting tea to the affected region. In addition to reducing inflammation, this hastens the healing process.

Topical Uses of Herbs

Several topical herbal remedies can be used directly on insect bites, in addition to herbal beverages and balms.

Applying aloe vera, which is well-known for its calming and cooling qualities, to bites can provide immediate relief. Crushed plantain leaves can be applied to the affected region to help lessen irritation and inflammation.

Because essential oils have anti-inflammatory and antibacterial properties, they can be applied to bites gently when diluted with carrier oil, such as eucalyptus and tea tree oil.

Herbal remedies for insect bites provide a comprehensive method of symptom relief and healing.

These remedies use the power of nature to relieve the pain produced by insect bites, whether through the use of anti-inflammatory beverages, calming balms, or focused topical therapies.

CHAPTER FOUR

HERBAL PREVENTATIVE REMEDIES

Herbs have long been used to treat and prevent a wide range of illnesses, including poisoning and insect stings. The likelihood of running into these problems when participating in outdoor activities can be considerably decreased by incorporating preventative herbal measures. Using natural insect and danger repellents is an important part of the process.

Organic Repellents

Some herbs are naturally insect repellent, thus they are a great addition to formulas meant to ward against bites. Citronella, which is obtained from lemongrass, is a well-known organic bug deterrent. It works as an efficient repellent because its potent aroma covers up smells that draw insects. Other essential oils with insect-repelling qualities include eucalyptus, peppermint, and lavender. They offer a natural defense against bites and can be added to herbal treatments in a variety of forms, including sprays, lotions, and diffusers.

Moreover, topical applications of herbal mixtures like neem, citronella, and tea tree oil can form a barrier of defense. Neem's antibacterial and antifungal qualities aid in soothing skin in addition to keeping insects away. Incorporating these plants into repellent mixtures guarantees a comprehensive strategy to avoid insect stings and possible toxicity exposure.

Herbal Remedies For Outdoor Pursuits

People who participate in outdoor activities run the danger of being ill from poisoning and getting bitten by insects.

For such situations, herbal remedies are crucial to bringing about fast alleviation.

Because of its calming qualities, aloe vera can be administered topically to reduce the pain that comes with insect bites. Its calming properties aid in lowering irritation and inflammation.

Moreover, a traditional cure for pest bites is to apply crushed plantain leaves. Plantain leaves have antibacterial and anti-inflammatory qualities that aid in healing.

Additionally, for its relaxing and anti-inflammatory properties, a poultice prepared from calendula and chamomile can be applied on bites.

Jewelweed is a natural remedy for poison ivy and oak exposures; it is applied topically to counteract the symptoms.

Jewelweed sap relieves irritation and inflammation by neutralizing the irritants found in poison ivy and oak.

By incorporating these herbal remedies into outdoor activities, poison, and bug bites can be prevented and treated naturally and comprehensively.

To have a safe and successful experience with herbal treatments, it is necessary to know individual sensitivities and certain plants and their properties.

CHAPTER FIVE

HERBS USED IN CONVENTIONAL MEDICARE

Since ancient times, herbs have been used extensively in traditional medicine as all-natural cures for a wide range of illnesses. Herbs have been used for centuries to cure poisoning and bug bites, offering relief and healing in the process. Gaining knowledge about the cultural customs and historical viewpoints related to these plants helps us appreciate how effective they are in handling similar circumstances.

Historical Angles

Herbs have long been used to cure poisoning and bug stings going back thousands of years. Native American tribes and traditional healers frequently used the local flora to mitigate the negative effects of poisonous plants or venomous bites. Ancient literature that documents herbal medicines attests to the long-standing acknowledgment of particular plants' therapeutic qualities.

Through trial and error, herbal mixtures were created, and knowledge was passed down through the generations. Ancient societies fostered a strong bond between nature and medicinal techniques by realizing the value of specific herbs in reducing the effects of poisons. Some herbs, like yarrow and echinacea, were well known for their ability to treat poison-related problems, while others, including plantain, comfrey, and calendula, were frequently used to relieve insect bites.

Cultural Customs

Due to the influence of their native plants and geographic location, various civilizations have different views on using herbs to treat poisoning and bug bites.

Based on their knowledge of regional herbs and their medicinal properties, traditional healers throughout the world created specialized treatments.

The spiritual significance associated with natural remedies is reflected in the frequent inclusion of these herbs in rituals and ceremonies that are part of cultural customs.

Certain herbs are employed not only for their therapeutic benefits but also for their symbolic meaning of warding off evil spirits connected to poisonous encounters.

In certain societies, these herbs are revered. The use of herbs in cultural rituals emphasizes the all-encompassing attitude to health that is characteristic of many traditional societies.

Comprehending the traditional use of plants for treating poisoning and bug bites is essential to recognize the variety of herbal treatments found throughout the world.

The wisdom that has been passed down through the ages not only protects traditional medical practices but also advances the continuous study of herbal remedies in modern settings. We obtain a thorough understanding of herbs' function in traditional medicine for treating poisoning and bug bites as we delve into the historical and cultural aspects of them.

CHAPTER SIX

HERBAL SOLUTIONS IN ACTION: CASE STUDIES

This section includes several real-world case studies of people who successfully treated poisoning and bug bites with herbal treatments. Every case study offers a thorough description of the particular circumstance, the herbal medicine that was applied, and the results that were seen. These stories provide powerful illustrations of the possible efficacy of herbal remedies.

Herbs For Exposure To Poisonous Plants

Some plants can irritate the skin or cause allergic responses when touched. This section's case studies highlight situations in which people came into contact with toxic plants and were able to successfully lessen their effects by employing herbal remedies.

The highlighted herbs, how they are applied, and the outcomes that are seen all add to a thorough knowledge of herbal therapies.

Poisonous Bite: Using Herbs To Reduce Toxic Effects

Serious effects can result from venomous bites from snakes, spiders, and other species. This section of the essay examines situations in which people sought solace from venomous bites by using herbal treatments.

The particular plants used, how they were prepared, and how the symptoms were subsequently relieved are all described in detail to demonstrate the possible advantages of herbal therapies.

Herbal Treatments for Insect Bite Itching and Swelling

Although they are typically not fatal, common bug bites can result in discomfort and allergic reactions. This section's case studies highlight people who used herbal treatments to effectively reduce swelling and itching brought on by insect bites.

The choice of plants, how they are applied, and the overall reduction in symptoms all add to a comprehensive understanding of herbal remedies.

Success Stories: References And Extended Results

This section gathers testimonies and success stories from people who have used herbal remedies in their first aid routines.

These personal accounts offer an expanded viewpoint on the enduring efficacy of herbal medicines, highlighting the enduring advantages and favorable consequences encountered by individuals who have integrated herbs into their strategy for treating poisoning and insect bites.

Examining case studies and success stories highlights how effective herbal remedies may be for treating poisoning and bug bites. Although individual reactions may differ, the aggregate body of research described in this article indicates that herbal treatments can be beneficial for both general well-being and first aid.

CHAPTER SEVEN

HERBAL DIET FOR GENERAL WELL-BEING

Adopting a herbal lifestyle benefits general health as well as the treatment of certain ailments. This section promotes a holistic approach to health and well-being by highlighting the incorporation of herbal practices into everyday life.

Using Herbs In Everyday Living

There are helpful hints and instructions on how to include herbs in everyday practices. This section covers a variety of methods to incorporate herbs into daily living pleasantly and naturally, from making herbal teas to adding particular plants to meals.

Nutrition And Herbal Diet

Supporting the body's innate ability to fight infections is mostly dependent on diet. This section delves into an herbal approach to nutrition and diet, emphasizing foods and herbs that can help prevent and treat fungal infections like athlete's foot.

People might strengthen their immune systems and improve their general health by switching to a herbal diet.

For individuals looking for herbal remedies to treat fungal infections like athlete's foot, this guide provides an extensive resource.

People can take charge of their skin health and resilience by being aware of the conditions, appreciating the benefits of herbal therapies, and adopting an herbal lifestyle.

CHAPTER EIGHT

TREATING HERBS AS AN INGREDIENT

Growing therapeutic herbs in one's garden is a fulfilling and all-encompassing approach to well-being. You can sustainably obtain natural medications, such as those that work well for treating poisoning and insect stings, by cultivating your medical herb garden. We'll look at how to grow and use medicinal herbs to treat these particular issues in this section.

Developing Your Herbal Medicine Garden

Planting a therapeutic herb garden is the first step towards using herbal remedies for poisoning and insect stings.

It's important to choose the correct herbs and create an environment that supports their growth. Popular remedies for poisoning and insect bites include plantain, aloe vera, calendula, and lavender. These herbs can help lessen the effects of bites and stings because of their anti-inflammatory, antiseptic, and calming qualities.

Comprehending the distinct requirements of every herb is vital for accomplished gardening. Take into account elements like water requirements, soil makeup, and sunlight.

For example, lavender likes slightly alkaline soil and regular watering, whereas aloe vera grows best in well-draining soil with lots of sunlight. You can make sure that the herbs in your garden fulfill their therapeutic potential by designing them to suit these requirements.

A flourishing herb garden requires regular upkeep. Plant health is influenced by pruning, weeding, and giving them the right nutrition.

This increases their potency and guarantees a plentiful and sustainable supply of herbs for a range of medical uses.

Gathering And Preserving Herbs

Timely harvesting of herbs is essential to maintaining their therapeutic qualities. varied herbs require varied timing, therefore it's important to learn the exact instructions for each plant. Since the active substances in the plants are concentrated during their flowering stage, harvesting is often best done during this time.

To keep your picked herbs effective, it's important to dry and store them properly. One popular technique is to air dry the herbs by hanging them in a dry, well-ventilated place. To preserve the essential oils, make sure the drying procedure takes place out of direct sunlight. After drying, place the herbs in airtight jars and keep them somewhere cold and dark. This preserves their effectiveness and gives you access to a ready source for making herbal treatments.

Developing a therapeutic herb garden provides an eco-friendly and organic way to treat poisoning and insect stings. Through comprehension of the distinct requirements of every herb, use of appropriate farming methods, and proficiency in the processes of harvesting and preserving, you can fully utilize herbal treatments to advance health and wellness.

CHAPTER NINE

SAFETY MEASUREMENTS AND ASSESSMENT

It is critical to protect the health and safety of people who have been bitten by toxins or insects. It is important to emphasize that in cases of severe illness, it is imperative to seek emergency medical treatment before experimenting with herbal medicines. Herbal remedies can provide some relief for minor instances, but in other cases, immediate medical attention is necessary. Always err on the side of caution, particularly in situations where it's unclear how serious the bite is or what kind of reaction it might cause.

When To Get Expert Assistance

It's critical to recognize the warning signs and know when to seek expert medical assistance. A more serious condition that needs to be attended to right once may be indicated by severe allergic responses, breathing difficulties, facial or throat swelling, and excruciating pain. When this happens, speed is the key, and using herbal medicines alone might not be enough. Prioritizing the patient's health and contacting medical professionals as soon as possible are essential.

Interactions Between Herbal Medicine And Conventional Medicine

It's important to take into account any possible interactions with prescription medications when investigating herbal remedies for poisoning and insect bites. Certain herbs have the potential to worsen pre-existing medical issues or cause drug interactions. Before using herbal therapies, it is best to speak with a healthcare provider, particularly if the patient is already taking medication or has a history of health issues. This preventive measure guarantees a thorough comprehension of how herbal remedies might work in conjunction with or contrast with traditional medical treatments.

Herbs For Insect And Poison Bite

Many plants found in nature have been shown to provide calming and restorative effects on poisoning and insect bites. In milder events, these cures can provide relief and aid in the healing process, but they may not be a suitable substitute for professional medical care in more severe cases.

Plantain: The antibacterial and anti-inflammatory qualities of the common plantain leaf are well-known. Insect bite pain and swelling can be lessened by directly applying a poultice prepared from crushed plantain leaves to the afflicted region.

Calendula: Calendula is an excellent remedy for skin irritations brought on by insect bites because of its calming and anti-inflammatory qualities. You can apply a calendula-infused cream or ointment topically to aid with healing and ease discomfort.

Aloe Vera: Known for its soothing and anti-inflammatory qualities, aloe vera gel helps ease the pain and irritation brought on by insect bites. Recovering faster may be possible if freshly extracted aloe vera gel is applied to the affected area.

Chamomile: Chamomile has anti-inflammatory and sedative qualities that make it useful for treating bug bite pain topically or as a compress. You can lessen redness and irritation by applying a lotion or compress laced with chamomile.

Lavender: The calming and antibacterial properties of lavender essential oil are well known. Pain relief and infection prevention can be achieved by diluting of a few drops of lavender oil in a carrier oil and application to the affected area.

Security And Efficiency

Herbal medicines have certain limitations, yet they can be helpful for minor poisonings and bug stings. Severe responses or venomous animal bites may necessitate emergency medical care. Furthermore, different people will respond differently to herbal remedies, and outcomes might not happen right away. Applying herbal treatments consistently and keeping an eye out for any negative reactions are crucial for safe and efficient use.

Using Herbs In Everyday Living

Taking preventive action is essential for reducing the chance of poisoning and bug bites. Including some herbs in your routine can provide extra protection or serve as a natural deterrent.

Citronella: Citronella has a reputation for keeping insects away. Citronella oil can be applied topically or used in diffusers and candles to help provide a barrier against mosquitoes and other biting insects.

Mint: Mint leaves have a natural insect-repellant effect when crushed or used as essential oil. An environment free of bugs can be achieved by growing mint around outdoor living areas or by utilizing items infused with mint.

Eucalyptus: The potent aroma of eucalyptus oil can keep mosquitoes away. Applying a mixture of eucalyptus and carrier oil on exposed skin will help deter mosquitoes and other biting insects.

Herbal remedies for bugs and poisonous bites can be a great help for minor events, relieving itching, swelling, and pain. But in severe circumstances, it's important to prioritize getting expert medical attention and understand the limitations of natural therapies. Effective and responsible use of herbal remedies requires observance of safety guidelines, prompt consultation with medical specialists, and knowledge of possible interactions with conventional medications. A comprehensive strategy to reduce the danger of poisoning and insect bites might include implementing preventive measures, such as adding insect-repelling herbs into daily living.

FINAL VERDICT

As we conclude our investigation into herbal remedies for fungal infections and athlete's foot, it is important to summarize the most important learnings. This final section reviews the herbal medicines covered in the book and offers a comprehensive overview of their uses and advantages. It is recommended that readers incorporate this herbal knowledge into their daily lives to achieve a comprehensive and long-lasting approach to wellness.

Recap Of Herbal Remedies

For those looking for a fast overview of the cures covered, a brief synopsis of the herbal remedies is a useful resource. Important herbs, their characteristics, and applications for treating fungal infections and athlete's feet are highlighted in this section. Readers can quickly include these treatments in their wellness regimens by summarizing the herbal possibilities.

Access To Herbal Knowledge

In this book, empowerment through knowledge is the main focus. Giving readers a thorough understanding of herbal remedies empowers them to make knowledgeable decisions regarding their health. This section highlights the significance of actively participating in one's health and empowers people to confidently investigate herbal substitutes.

Adopting the knowledge of herbal remedies can result in a more natural and balanced approach to health. Herbs can be used in daily life to promote overall health, manage fungal infections, and avoid athlete's foot, among other things. This can lead to a more fulfilling and active lifestyle.